Words of Wisdom®

Nursing

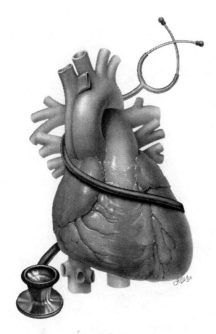

Ex libris

Nurse _____

Edition 1

authorHOUSE®

AuthorHouse™
1663 Liberty Drive
Bloomington, IN 47403
www.authorhouse.com
Phone: 1-800-839-8640

First published by AuthorHouse 3/17/2011

ISBN: 978-1-4567-3182-3 (e)
ISBN: 978-1-4567-3183-0 (sc)

Library of Congress Control Number: 2011902146

Printed in the United States of America

Any people depicted in stock imagery provided by Thinkstock are models,
and such images are being used for illustrative purposes only.
Certain stock imagery © Thinkstock.

This book is printed on acid-free paper.

Words of Wisdom®

Nursing

Edition 1

Laurence D. Pfeiffer, DDS, MD
Resident
Department of Oral and Maxillofacial Surgery
University of Texas Southwestern Medical Center
Dallas, Texas

Contributor

John N. Phelan, PhD
Assistant Professor of Anatomy
Department of Cell Biology
University of Texas Southwestern Medical Center
Dallas, Texas

Illustrations and Design

Lindsay Oksenberg, MA
www.lindsayoksenberg.com
Medical Illustrator
Department of Geriatrics
University of Texas Southwestern Medical Center
Dallas, Texas

Consultants

Mary Fisher, RN
Clinical Nurse
Parkland Health and Hospital System
Dallas, Texas

Kynyatta Green, RN, BS
Clinical Nurse
Parkland Health and Hospital System
Dallas, Texas

Sharla Turner, RN, BSN
Nurse Manager
Parkland Health and Hospital System
Dallas, Texas

Carolina Weseman, RN, BSN
Clinical Nurse
Parkland Health and Hospital System
Dallas, Texas

Sara Wilensky RN, BSN
Clinical Nurse
Parkland Health and Hospital System
Dallas, Texas

To my mom and dad

Contents

Introduction

This book is unique. There is no plot, no "situation", no protagonist. There is no profound problem to solve. This book is a collection of words of wisdom by professionals who are exceptionally skilled, highly trained, and vital to the medical and heathcare community. These are nurses and they have inspiring and important messages for those in the profession, as well as others in the medical and healthcare field. Collectively the nurses whose words of wisdom are printed here have hundreds of years of education and clinical or research experience. Many have been pioneers in the field of nursing.

When I first set out to develop this book, I knew I wanted a broad representation of nurses to share their "words of wisdom" with the rest of us. I invited nurses to participate based on what I knew to be their commitment and contribution to the field, their research, and their academic achievements. Those interested responded and their contributions are contained here.

I am grateful that so many talented and gifted nurses saw the value and importance of this project to take time out to share their advice and experience.

This book is the second of several medical, nursing, and dental specialty books. I hope more nurses will participate in future editions and join those who chose to be in this, the first, *Words of Wisdom: Nursing*.

To all of you who contributed your nursing wisdom, I express my sincere admiration and gratitude.

Thank you for your efforts, your commitment to the profession, and the care you give your patients.

For those long in the nursing field, just entering it, or even just considering it, I believe you will find their "words of wisdom" an invaluable resource in your journey.

LAURENCE D. PFEIFFER, DDS, MD
Resident
Department of Oral and Maxillofacial Surgery
University of Texas Southwestern Medical Center
Dallas, Texas

My Wisdom

Wash your hands. Hand washing is probably one of the most important rituals that all healthcare providers can possibly do, not only for the patient's sake but for yours as well. Keeping your hands clean is one of the most essential ways to prevent the spread of infection and illness.

Treat all patients as if they were your family. If you have ever been on the receiving end of vital medical information you will understand.

If you do not know the answer to a question, find someone who does or look it up.

Be warm with your presentation. Never be afraid to make your patients laugh.

Always protect your eyes with a face shield or some equivalent. Blood and debris are sneaky and they can find themselves anywhere at any time.

Don't let a day go by without telling your parents you appreciate all they have done for you and most importantly that you love them. Life changes very quickly when you least expect it.

Protect yourself from needle sticks. Pay attention to where the needle is and where your hands are. Know the number to call in case of a needle stick injury.

Smoking cessation for all tobacco users is an absolute must. Be persistent and be honest with them. If there are any guarantees in this world it is that smoking will kill you.

These are just a few of my words of wisdom that have helped me as a dental and medical student and now as an oral and maxillofacial surgery resident. I learned many of these bits of wisdom by watching and working alongside nurses. I am fortunate to have had nurses assist me with running codes, managing infected wounds, starting difficult IVs, and assisting with everyday patient management. I have been saved many times by diligent nurses and they have been instrumental in my becoming a better oral and maxillofacial surgeon.

The field of nursing has been built and shaped by outstanding and innovative nurses like those who share their words of nursing wisdom here. Many of these participating nurses devote their time and talents to research, many have written journal articles and text books that are used on a daily basis, many train other nurses, and each and every one of them have devoted themselves to caring for patients and have helped evolve the medical specialty of nursing into the vibrant, diverse, and challenging field that it is today. It would be amazing to have the opportunity to sit down with each of these nurses in person and absorb as much of their knowledge as possible, to hear their stories and their words of wisdom. But we all know that this is impossible because we are all in different locations around the country. Let this book be a way for you to have a brief meeting with these amazing nurses. I think you will find, as I have in my own medical education and practice, and in compiling this book, that they have much wisdom to share.

LAURENCE D. PFEIFFER, DDS, MD
Resident
Department of Oral and Maxillofacial Surgery
University of Texas Southwestern Medical Center
Dallas, Texas

Anatomy Plates

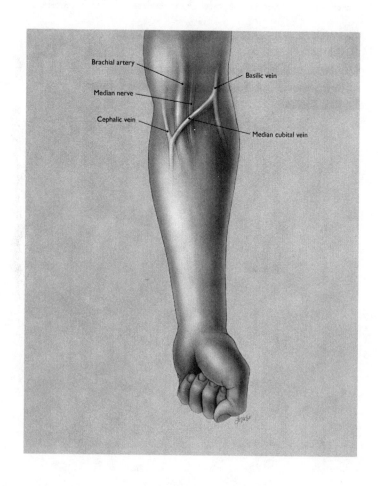

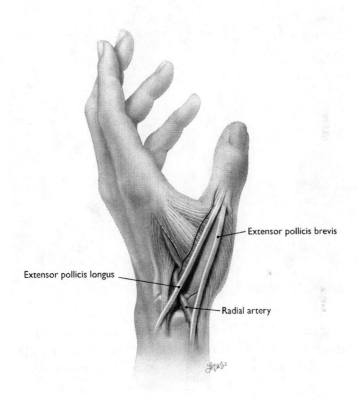

Extensor pollicis brevis

Extensor pollicis longus

Radial artery

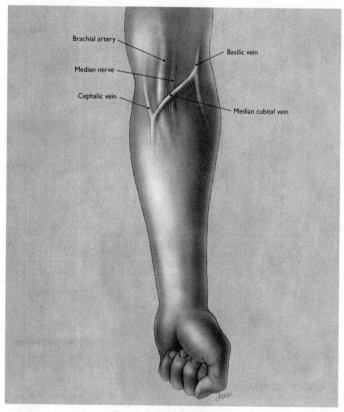

Fig. 1 Ante cubital region

The median cubital vein connects two superficial veins of the arm, the cephalic and basilic, in the cubital fossa, the region opposite the elbow. The most common configuration among these veins is the H-shaped pattern shown in the accompanying drawing. The median cubital vein is a popular target for venipuncture due to its size, its proximity to the skin, and the fact that it is infrequently absent. Additionally, it tends to stay in place while being penetrated with a needle because of its tight connections to deeper veins. The cephalic vein in the arm, meanwhile, is less tightly connected to its tributaries and is likely to shift away from a needle when venipuncture is attempted.

The basilic vein is a less desirable candidate for venipuncture because it is closely accompanied in the arm and forearm by a cutaneous nerve which could be damaged by the needle; the same is true for the cephalic vein in the forearm. Also, accidentally puncturing the posterior side of the basilic vein could damage the closely associated brachial artery. Damage to the underlying brachial artery and median nerve during puncture of the median cubital vein is unlikely because the vein is separated from the artery and nerve by a tough fascial sheet, the bicipital aponeurosis, which resists penetration.

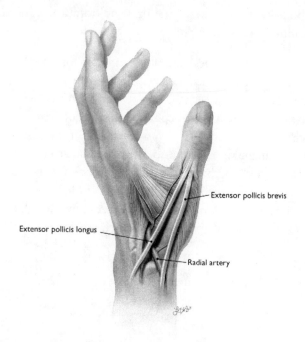

Extensor pollicis brevis

Extensor pollicis longus

Radial artery

Fig. 2 Anatomical snuff box

A patient's heart rate can be measured by lightly pressing two fingertips against the anterior surface of the wrist at the base of the thumb. This action compresses the radial artery against the underlying radius and allows detection of that artery's pulse. A good palpable landmark to assist in locating the radial artery is the flexor carpi radialis, as the artery lies just lateral to the tendon of this muscle. Distal to this point on the wrist the radial artery passes deep into the anatomical snuff box, which is bordered by the tendons of the extensor pollicis longus and brevis and the abductor pollicis longus. While the radial artery is not as close to the surface in the anatomical snuff box as it is in the wrist, its pulse may still be palpated here.

    " I am thirty-four years a nurse this year. It has been a long
       and tremendously meaningful journey in which I have
       grown to be a far better person because of the people
I have cared for. Some of my moments of greatest learning
and greatest connection in life have been with patients. My
most meaningful gifts have come from drawing close to
patients in their moments of greatest vulnerability. In those
moments, the periphery fades and the essence of what is
most important and most true in life comes to light.

First and foremost in my career, there was Ernie who had a
spinal fusion at Boston Children's Hospital and required a
good deal of care post-operatively in halo-femoral traction.
I was a young nurse at the time and the initial sight of
Ernie face down on the striker frame with large screws in
his skull caught my breath. His voice invited me to move
past my apprehensions and draw closer. This young man,
in the most compromising of positions, needed my help
and my compassion. He made a few jokes to ease my initial
trepidations, and slowly I grew to know Ernie very well.
Between wound care and intravenous infusions, I met the
young man who had spent many months over many years
in city hospitals. He spoke about his history of twenty-
plus surgeries and the stress it had brought to his family,
especially his mom. Ernie was a wonderfully complex
young man just turning twenty: vulnerable and strong,
at-risk and resilient, a patient and a teacher of nurses. He
was an amazing human being who needed the best I could

give so I gave that. I summoned all of the science and all of the art of nursing that I had been schooled to give and slowly Ernie grew stronger and more independent again. Having been disabled his entire life, Ernie shared his hopes and fears about becoming a young adult and transitioning to independent living. Somewhere in between assessments and interventions, I learned who Ernie really was and who he hoped to be. And as I listened, I grew stronger from witnessing his courage and fortitude. He was sharing from deep within and I was the recipient of some amazing gifts there for the taking.

The lessons from Ernie have been life-long for me. Listen carefully to who is on the other side of your care. Take the time to hear their struggle and quest for finding meaning in the experience. Give your best from your mind and your heart. The patients can feel your intentions in your eye contact and your touch. Be gentle and strong. Be honest and share the steps of your care with them. Earn their trust the old fashioned way: by seeing their need for dignity and by caring for each person thoughtfully and intentionally. Nurses are given the privilege of sharing some of the most vulnerable moments in a person's life: birth and death and all points in between. Respect that privilege and honor it. In that trust is something that borders on sacred. It has depth and meaning far beyond the next dressing change. Have the courage to enter that space with the highest level of respect and nobility. When you bring your best, the return on investment far outweighs the initial deposit. You become witness to the human spirit under great challenge and in a few moments, you will see the purest forms of human triumph and despair. You will journey with families down some of the darkest roads and be surprised by some of the sources of light.

I am reminded of the story of the velveteen rabbit. Yes, after thirty-four years of nursing, my hair is thinner and I am a bit ragged from the wear. But I am a far better person from the connections with my patients, the insights gained, the warmth shared and the tears shed. I cannot regret one day and I know when I am an old lady rocking on that porch that I will close my eyes and fill with all that has been given back to me: the riches of the human spirit and the treasures of the souls touched."

CYNTHIA C. ADAMS, RN, MS, EdD
Director of Nursing
Capital Community College
Hartford, CT
Expertise:
Hospice
Nursing Education
Nursing Leadership
Education:
Simmons College, Bachelors in Nursing
Boston College, Masters of Science in Community
    Health Nursing
University of Hartford, Doctorate in Educational Leadership

❝ Whenever a patient's personality has changed, do not assume there is no physiological underlying reason. Think of the brain as the 'spoiled brat' of the body. A change of level of consciousness is usually the first indicator that the patient's status has changed. Rule out possible precipitating factors such as: hypoxia, adverse reaction to a medication, toxic levels of a medication, etc. In a nutshell: pleasant, oriented patients do not suddenly become irritable, confused patients without an underlying cause."

Irma G. Aguilar, RN, PhD
Associate Professor
Tarrant Community College Nursing Department
Fort Worth, TX
Expertise:
Mental Health
Education:
University of Texas at San Antonio Health Science Center (PhD)

❝ It is not how smart you are, but how smart you want to be. You can do anything you want; you just have to be persistent. Always set goals and look to the future. Looking toward the future must include reflecting upon the past, synthesis of perceptions, and connecting with what is known. Explore all possibilities; accept challenges, both professionally and personally."

"Learning does not end with college; as nurses we must continue to learn new things, expand our minds, and reach beyond where we are today. As Henry Ford once said, 'Anyone who stops learning is old, whether at twenty or eighty. Anyone who keeps learning stays young. The greatest thing in life is to keep your mind young.'"

Pamela L. Alderman, RN, MSN, ABD

Dean for Career and Technical Programs
Southern West Virginia Community and Technical College
Mount Gay, WV

Expertise:

Accreditation
Associate Degree Nursing
Curriculum Development
Emergency Nursing
Grant Writing
Higher Education
Leadership
Regulation
Stress Management

Education:

Southern West Virginia Community and Technical College (ASN)
West Virginia University (BSN, MSN)

" Be true to yourself and always be proud to be a NURSE! It is the most beautiful and rewarding profession. It is exhausting, challenging, and frustrating at times, but with strength and tenacity we will gain respect and power that will lead us into the next phase of independent practice. Never say, 'I'm just the nurse.' You are the heart and soul of health care. No other professional gives so much and understands so much all at once about science, art, family, social systems, and the human spirit. Last, be kind and support all those who work alongside of you. Nurses need to support and encourage one another. Be kind to physicians, aides, dieticians, housekeepers, and all those who work with you. A small effort to be interested and friendly will provide you with a network of friends to keep for many years. Patients and families will know when you are sincere, competent, and caring. Show them every day how to become better at taking care of each other. We are the most respected profession. Let's make sure we never lose that status."

KIM SIARKOWSKI AMER, PhD, RN
Associate Professor in Nursing
DePaul University
Chicago, IL
Expertise:
Theory in Nursing
Quality and Safety
Child Adaptation to Chronic Illness
Education:
St. Mary's College

❝ Nursing makes a difference. To be a good nurse, you have to have a passion for excellence in everything that you do. Everything you do as a nurse affects someone who is the most important person in the world to his/her family. All of these people are counting on you. Every one of these people need, want, and deserve your very best all the time. Be there for them with all of the knowledge and skill that nursing has to offer. This means that you are always learning and always looking for a better way.

You will save lives, change lives, and the doing of this will change you in ways you never imagined. Cherish your colleagues who stretch you to always go the distance, help you learn how to do things better, and support you during the best and worst of times. Be that colleague to others. When you are tired and your light is flickering, turn to your colleagues who will relight that flame for you.

Love the unlovable and find the good in every person. Every person has value and more than deserves our care, compassion, and love. Caring for people during the worst times in their lives is a privilege that few are allowed to have. Be thankful that your patients trusted you with their worst moments, greatest fears, and most challenging problems. The angriest person in the room is always the most frightened. Help him/her to feel safe. Human dignity always wants to flourish. You are the gardener who insures that it can.

Seek solutions to the unsolvable problems. Even one step toward a solution is better than inaction. Problems are like coins. When you cannot find a solution, turn the coin over and try a different way.

Never blink or look away when wrong things are happening because the reason you 'happen' to be there is to see that they do not happen. In life's game of tag, you will always be 'it'. Nursing is the safety net in health care.

Love this profession because you have been given a great legacy. Love what you do and find joy in the small things. The great things will find you. While you will believe that you are just one person who cannot possibly change the world, know that what you do may mean the world to just one person. Nurses change the world one day at a time, one patient at a time, and often just one minute at a time."

L. Antoinette (Toni) Bargagliotti, DNSc, RN, ANEF

Professor
Loewenberg School of Nursing
University of Memphis
Memphis, TN

Expertise:
Critical Care
Nursing Curriculum
Health Policy
Nursing Theory
Leadership
Nursing Administration
Nursing Education

Education:
University of California at San Francisco – DNSc
University of California at San Francisco – MSN
University of Tennessee Center for the Health Sciences- BSN
Tacoma General Hospital – Diploma

❝ The physician with whom you are consulting will always ask you the one question you didn't ask the patient!"

"Words of wisdom I learned from my former dean, Joan Hrubetz, PhD, RN, who is now deceased:

'I believe you have a responsibility to be passionate about something outside of yourself and your family. Set your sights high. Search your soul until you find a cause about which you feel passionately; then contribute to that cause. Do not deprive yourself of the things you've worked so hard to get. Rather, enrich yourself by reaching beyond the boundaries of your life to touch the lives of those less fortunate than you. Also, remember your responsibilities to yourself. Read poetry. Take pleasure in children. Laugh often and gleefully. Listen to Mozart. Say, 'I love you' often and sincerely. Occasionally dance until dawn. Cry when you must—and share your tears. Find meaning in death and in life. Now go out and change the world. You can, you know.'"

MARY LEE BARRON, PhD, APRN, FNP-BC
Director, MSN and DNP Programs
School of Nursing
Saint Louis University
St. Louis, MO
Expertise:
Teaching NP Students
Womens' Health Clinical Issues
Education:
Saint Louis University

" When I was a brand new nurse on orientation, the very first patient I took care of gave me great advice just days before he passed. He said, 'You just have to listen. If you always listen, you'll always be ok.'

Listen to your coworkers. If you don't have the answer, someone else will. Leave all of your pocket guides that you stuffed your nursing school uniforms with at home. You will have multiple real-life resources that can answer any question quicker than you can look it up. You will spend more time with them than with your real family and friends, and once you build each others' trust, you will never feel scared or alone at work.

Listen to your patients: More times than not, they are right. If they tell you they've never seen the pill you are giving them, they probably haven't. Don't chalk it up to 'old age' or 'a generic brand,' because chances are, you will be wrong. *They* will be right.

Listen to your doctors: They are a wealth of knowledge and you will learn more from them in a conversation than you'll even realize you learned. Please note: This does not apply to interns during the month of July. In this case, they will often be listening to you, so speak up. Be quick to question. Multiple lives have been saved by nurses catching errors that new doctors make. If an order that is written seems wrong to you, it probably is. Call a coworker, pharmacist, or supervisor if you need to. Just because an order is written by a doctor does not mean you need to carry it through. This is your license and most importantly your patient's life on the line.

Listen to yourself: Follow your instincts and be confident in the choices you make. Chances are there is a reason you made that choice. The nurse's instinct is a very powerful feeling that will hit you at the perfect time, exactly when you need it. You won't have to ask or think. You will just act. And at the end of the day the chances are, you will be right."

LINDSAY BROWN, BSN
Registered Nurse
Memorial Sloan Kettering Cancer Center
New York, NY
Expertise:
Oncology – Leukemia and Lymphoma
Education:
Seton Hall University, Accelerated Second Degree BSN

" Encourage those who are timid. Take tender care of those who are weak. Be always caring and patient with everyone." (1 Thess. 5:14, paraphrased)

GLORIA ANN BROWNING, PhD, MSN, RN
Nursing Faculty
University of Tennessee at Martin
Martin, TN
Expertise:
Medical-Surgical Nursing
Community Health Nursing
Education:
Austin Peay State University (BSN)
University of Phoenix (MSN)
University of New Mexico (PhD)

“ If you can't see the humor in nursing, please leave."

EILEEN BRUNER, MS, BSN, RN-BC
Instructor
South Dakota State University College of Nursing
Brookings, SD
Expertise:
Gerontology
Community Health
Education:
Mount Marty College (BSN)
South Dakota State University (MS)

" Nursing practice: Don't rush into a position for a paycheck, match it to your philosophy of care and your heart."

"Physical exams: The best instruments you can use are your five senses."

"Patient care: Respect and listen to every woman as if she were your mother or sister."

"Obstetric Nursing; It is a privilege and an honor to assist in the birth of a child; don't let it get to be routine."

"Newborns: The best place for a newborn to transition is skin to skin with his/her mom or dad, not the infant warmer."

"Birth: The physiology of birth is a normal process, don't mess with Mother Nature unless absolutely necessary."

"Nursing Students: Treat nursing students with respect; at some time and place they may become your supervisor."

Barbara Camune, CNM, WHNP-BC, DrPH, FACNM

Clinical Associate Professor
Staff Midwife, AVIVA Women's Health & Midwifery Care
Midwifery and Women's Health Nurse Practitioner Programs
University of Illinois at Chicago
Chicago, IL

Expertise:
Women's Health Care
Newborn Care

Education:
Northern Illinois University (BSN)
University of Texas at Galveston (MSN & Post Masters' Midwifery)
University of Texas Health Science Center Houston
School of Public Health (DrPH)

In order to create a sustainable caring practice, self care must be practiced by the nurse. Unfortunately, the idea of caring for oneself is under-emphasized amongst the rigors of pre-licensure nursing education and in the workplace, so it often is up to the individual nurse to create their own self-care modalities and experiences. Self-care goes beyond addressing one's physical needs and delves into the realm of a spiritual-healing journey. Nurses who have the courage to undertake such a healing journey are better able to care for their patients in time of need and realize the historical spiritual roots of our practice as nurses, caring for those who are suffering and in need. I encourage all nurses to find ways to care for themselves everyday, and to share the journey with colleagues."

CAREY S. CLARK, RN, PhD

Assistant Professor
University of Maine
Augusta, ME
Expertise:
Caring in Nursing
Academia
Hospice
Community Health
Parish Nursing
Education:
Rio Hondo College
Excelsior College
California State University, Dominguez Hills

On Nursing Practice:

"Clinical care is the bread and butter of nursing; don't spread your butter too thinly or give all your bread away."

On Acute Illness in General:

"Take care of the patient not the monitor."

On Teaching:

"Learning after kindergarten can still be fun."

On Taking Care of Your Patient:

"Treat the patient and their family as you would like to be treated."

NANCY CREGO, PhD-C, MSN, RN, CCRN
Nursing Professor
Georgetown University
Washington, DC
Expertise:
Pediatric Sedation
Pediatric Acute Care
Education:
Barry University (BSN, MSN)
University of Virginia (PhD)

❝ I have been a practicing registered nurse for more than 30 years, most of those years in the hospital setting. While I do not pretend to know everything, I can summarize my best advice for success in this profession in 3 words: caring, commitment and compassion."

On caring:

"Remember always why you entered this profession in the first place: 'I want to be able to take care of people.' Nursing is both an art and a science but it is the act of caring which sets it apart so distinctly from all others."

On commitment:

"Commit yourself to lifelong learning by making it your personal and professional goal to learn one new fact or viewpoint every day you work with patients. Don't overlook the important lesson of learning from your mistakes. Perhaps the greatest lessons to be learned are those involving the courage of the human spirit. Patients in pain or faced with a grave prognosis who can still smile and say 'thank you, nurse' never fail to touch my heart which brings me to the most important advice for nursing........."

On compassion:

"Without compassion and empathy for those entrusted to your care, nursing is absolutely meaningless. There is no other profession for which this is so vital and believe me, the patient is the first to know when compassion is lacking."

ANNE CROSS, MS, RN, CNE
Clinical Faculty
University of Connecticut School of Nursing
Storrs, CT
Expertise:
Adult Medical-Surgical Nursing
Over 25 years of Acute Care Experience
8 years of Teaching Undergraduate Nursing Students
    at the University Level
Education:
Norwalk Hospital School of Nursing
University of Hartford (BSN)
University of Connecticut (MS in Nursing)

" If you work with a computer documentation program, don't let the computer run your work flow."

"You will know when you find a GREAT mentor. Learn everything you can from that person."

"It is true; what you learned in kindergarten is applied in the nursing profession. You do not have to like everyone you work with, but you do have an obligation to provide the best, safest patient care and your nursing degree means you are a professional. Treat others with respect and it is okay to agree to disagree. This means you have to communicate with each other, even if you do not like each other. Communicating with co-workers is crucial for patient care."

"Speak up when you make a mistake. This proves you have integrity and care about the care you are providing. Unfortunately, we are human and make them. Anyone who tells you they have not made a mistake is lying to you or is so self-centered that they do not know they have made the mistake. We learn from our mistakes and others learn from our mistakes."

"This is not an easy job but it is a very rewarding job. Treat every patient you have as if they were your family member and learn to speak up and be a patient advocate. It is a scary world for patients and they need you."

"It is ok to not know everything, but have enough courage to know that you don't know everything."

"HAVE FUN!!! Laugh A LOT! Cry if you need to!!"

DARLENE DOSS (ADKISON), MSN, RN
Clinical Educator
Clarian Arnett Health
Lafayette, IN
Expertise:
Medical-Surgical Nurse for 10 years
Adjunct Faculty for Indiana University School of Nursing
Adjunct Faculty for Purdue School of Nursing
Education:
William Carey University

" Sometimes it's hard to see the patient (and their needs) for the surrounding equipment, monitors and other accoutrements of hospital care."

KATHY DUNNE, RN, MSN, CNM, NP
Clinical Instructor
University of Illinois at Chicago College of Nursing
Chicago, IL
Expertise:
Midwifery
Maternal/Family Nursing
Education:
St. Xavier University in Chicago (BSN)
University of Illinois at Chicago College of Nursing (MS)

Remember that you only have one opportunity to make a 'first impression.' When you approach the bedside of the patient, remember that your competency, to a very large degree, will be judged by your professional comportment. Every patient wants to feel safe in your care and to believe that you are there because of the specialized knowledge and skills that you have as a professional nurse holding that license to practice. Look and behave like the nurse you would want to see approach your bedside or the bedside of someone you love. Remove the facial piercings and the tongue rings, cover the obvious tattoos and have a traditional hair color and style. Respect your audience and consider the circumstances of your meeting. This person is sick and is counting on you to take care of him and to be his advocate. Be kind, caring, empathetic, supportive and confidant in your knowledge and skills. If you always take a minute to reflect and put yourself in the place of the person in that bed and proceed to treat that patient accordingly, you will not go wrong."

Carol Eliadi, EdD, JD, APRN
Dean and Chief Nursing Officer
Massachusetts College of Pharmacy and Health Sciences
Boston, MA
Expertise:
Adult Nurse Practitioner
Legal Issues in Nursing and Healthcare
Education:
University of Massachusetts, Amherst MA

❝ The most important advice that I feel I can give to any nurse, but especially a new graduate, would be to have *confidence* in your ability as a nurse and to trust your gut instinct. As a nurse you have to be accountable for the actions and decisions you make and you need to make them confidently. This is not to say that you will not need guidance from other professionals, but it is a privilege to be a nurse and patients, families, doctors and other healthcare professionals will look to you for information that is crucial to your patients' survival and the care they receive at your institution. But, how do you do that?

It is not enough to know your patients' medical diagnoses. It is also crucial to understand their personal concerns which may affect their stay in the hospital and whether or not they will follow-up with treatment. Talk to your patients! Do not just simply ask them our standard questions about pain, hygiene habits and the focused assessment related to their reason for admission. Converse with them about what will make their stay better and how you can assure that they will continue to care for themselves when released from the hospital. When you truly know your patients and have knowledge of their needs, you will feel more confident and that will translate into better and safer patient care.❞

Marissa Elliott-Vizcarrondo,
MSN, RN, CNL
Registered Nurse
John Muir Behavioral Health Center
Adjunct Faculty
University of San Francisco
San Francisco, CA
Expertise:
Clinical Nurse Leader (CNL) Role Implementation
Education:
University of San Francisco

" On Student Nurses and Faculty:

Faculty shouldn't be working harder than students. If you find that you are working harder than they are to help them succeed, there is something wrong."

RUTH FIEDLER, EdD, PMHCNS-BC, CNE
Assistant Professor
Rush College of Nursing
Chicago, IL
Expertise:
Education
Psychiatric Nursing
Education:
West Suburban Hospital School of Nursing

" As a new nurse, be patient with yourself. Give yourself a year and then look back to see what you have accomplished and look forward to all that you have left to accomplish in the future."

"Care for all your patients like they were your family members. Show compassion even when it is hard."

"It is alright to cry with your patients and their families."

"Find a mentor that you trust after school and let him teach you."

DeLisa Flynn, RN, MSN, WHNP
ICU RN, Clinical Instructor
Ball State University and Indiana Wesleyan University
Muncie, IN
Expertise:
5.5 years ICU experience
4 years as critical care clinical instructor
Education:
Ball State University (RN)
Indiana University Purdue University Indianapolis
    (MSN, WHNP)

> **❝** Always treat every patient with the respect and care that you would want your own loved ones to receive."

VICKI FOX, ARNP, MSN, FNP
Outreach Clinician
Community Health Center of Snohomish County
Adjunct Faculty
Seattle University
Seattle, WA
Expertise:
Family Practice
Education:
University of Wisconsin Eau Claire (BSN)
University of Wisconsin Oshkosh (MSN)

❝ Advice to students about making clinical decisions:

When your instincts tell you something is wrong but it isn't what you learned in class, trust your instincts and report it. Remember, the patient hasn't read the textbook!"

JACQUELINE GUHDE, MSN, RN, CNS
Assistant Professor of Clinical Nursing
The University of Akron
Akron, OH
Expertise:
Medical-Surgical Nursing
Education:
Case Western Reserve University (BSN)
Kent State (MSN)

  It sounds really simple, but treat all patients as you would want your family to be treated. Eventually, you or your family will be on the receiving end of healthcare and you will know the helplessness that accompanies hospitalization. Over the years, I have seen so many nurses become overwhelmed with the demands of bedside nursing, i.e., short staffing, high acuity patients, etc. They become so frustrated at the lack of time and the overall stress of the job that they forget about the patient. Remember, it is not about us and how we are feeling. It is about the ones that need our care. Your frustration will affect everyone around you including your patient, the family, and your coworkers."

"Never label the individual by the diagnosis or disease. They are not 'the alcoholic,' 'the schizophrenic,' or 'the post-op hip replacement.' Learn their names. Everyone is more than just their diagnosis."

"Be kind to other nurses. Mentor new graduates. Listen to the sage advice of seasoned nurses. We must develop the new generation of nursing professionals and respect the generation that came before us. Everyone has something valuable to add to the profession."

"Be willing to admit you do not know something. If you are unable to ask questions or admit you made an error, you are dangerous."

"Be prepared for the emotional disillusionment you will

experience after you graduate from nursing school. No one ever tells you but the real healthcare environment is very different than what you experience in nursing school. In nursing school, your experiences are arranged and controlled by your professors; everything is idyllic and conducted in the manner in which it 'should be done.' However, once you are out in the 'real' world and on your own, you find everything is not as perfect. It might take a year or more to really settle in your new profession and find your niche, but be patient."

BETSY DI BENEDETTO GULLEDGE,
RN, MSN, PHDC
Nursing Instructor
Jacksonville State University
Jacksonville, AL
Fellow, Leadership in Education of Child Health Nursing
University of Alabama Birmingham
Birmingham, AL
Expertise:
Psychiatric/Mental Health Nursing
Child Health
Education:
Southern Union State Community College
Jacksonville State University
University of Alabama at Birmingham

❝ Our patients will tell us what they need and what is wrong with them, if we can only *truly* listen to them. This requires that we set aside our assumptions about them, our rapid-fire questions and our propensity to interrupt our patients. Quality patient care means letting the patient tell us their story fully."

VALERIE A. HART, EDD, PMHCNS, BC
Associate Professor
University of Southern Maine
Psychotherapist in Private Practice
Portland, ME

Expertise:
- Taught both undergraduate and graduate psychiatric nursing for over two decades.
- Research and scholarly interests include the role of advanced practice nurses as psychotherapists, women's mental health issues including infertility, and post-partum depression; teaching non-psychiatric advanced practice nurses about mental health issues, and patient communication.
- Her text, *Patient-Provider Communications: Caring to Listen* (2010) Jones & Bartlett, is the first book on patient communication written for advanced practice nurses.

Education:
Columbia University
Boston College

On becoming a nurse:

"Follow your heart, for nursing is a profession of the heart and the mind. Don't let anyone persuade you that you are too smart to be a nurse. Nurses need to be very smart. My dad was a physician and was pretty smart. His only sister was a nurse and she was smarter. As a public health nurse in Chicago in the 1920s, she had lunch with Jane Addams at Hull-House, took care of Al Capone's mother, and then spent most of her career as a school nurse and the only health care professional in a small town in Northern Minnesota, where she cared for and about everyone."

On nursing:

"Listening is more important than talking. Your patients will share their most private concerns and fears if you show that you are willing to listen to the whole story."

On nurse practitioners:

"This nursing role evolved out of public health nursing—that is no accident. Public health nurses know their patients, their patients' families, the neighborhoods in which their patients live and work and go to school. So do nurse practitioners, now the largest group of health care professionals providing primary care in the country."

JOELLEN W. HAWKINS, PHD,
WHNP-BC, FAAN, FAANP
Professor Emerita
William F. Connell School of Nursing
Boston College
Chestnut Hill, MA
Writer in Residence
Simmons College, Nursing Department
Boston, MA

Expertise:
Women's Health
Writing and Editing

Education:
Northwestern University (BSN)
Wesley Memorial Hospital School of Nursing (MS)
Boston College (PhD)

❝ On the Elderly:

You have to love them; one day you will be wearing 'diapers,' 'drooling,' and unable to get up.

On Practice:

Assess, ask why, question; you are the doctors' eyes and ears when they are not there.

On Being in School:

There are 2 C's in SuCCess.

On your Job:

It has to be a 'calling;' you will never be paid enough for what you do.

On Difficult Family:

Simply offer them a cup of coffee. You'd be amazed what a little caffeine can do for personalities.

On Patient Care:

Think about what makes you feel good; it is no different when you are lying in a hospital bed."

KAREN HILL, RN, BS, MN, PHD
Associate Professor
School of Nursing
Southeastern Louisiana University
Hammond, LA
Expertise:
Textbook Writing
Reviewing for Textbooks and NCLEX Questions
Pathophysiology
Pharmacology
Assessment
Cardiac Adult Nursing
Education:
Southeastern Louisiana University
Louisiana State University Medical School
University of New Orleans

❝ Dear Nursing Students,

Welcome into the wonderful world of nursing! Nursing is a challenging, complex, and very rewarding profession. I have been a registered nurse for over 35 years and a nursing professor for 13 years. My memories could fill many books. I have had the experience of working in ICU, CCU, ER, Medical and Surgical Nursing, and Mental Health, as well as in two nursing homes. You may ask which is my favorite area to work in, but I would not be able to narrow my choice. I have met so many unique individual persons in each area in which I have worked! My patients were from all age levels and each was at a different stage in their life journey. Nursing is not about having all of the high technological skills of an ICU nurse or about how many degrees that you have behind your name, although they are important. The true meaning of nursing comes from the amount of caring and compassion that you have inside of you. Listening with an open heart and open hands allows you to be ready to meet the most intimate needs of your patients. Each patient carries a story to tell that often bears a tremendous relationship to why they are currently ill. Broken families, lost loved ones, stress, economic hardships, limited education, social injustices, and loneliness are only a few of the real causes of a patient's illnesses. Being able to deliver holistic nursing is the true measure of a nurse. Social, emotional, psychological, physical, and spiritual needs must be met for each patient or client to become totally healed.

My advice to future nurses is to first 'believe in yourself' and your true self worth. Second, you must learn to trust in God who will give you the strength and wisdom that you need for every circumstance. You do not need to be at the top of your class with all of the highest academic grades on your exams. You need to have a dream of what you want to become as a person. Perseverance, commitment, creativity, and the power of 'never giving up' on what is important to you must be cultivated in every step of your own personal journey of becoming a professional nurse. Not only will your ability to advocate for a person come from your education and professional skills but it will be strengthened and guided by the amount of love and compassion that you have for the person that you are caring for! Nursing is not just a profession but it is a changing 'way of life' and will affect every aspect of your being. You will no longer be just a mother, father, sister, brother, or neighbor. You will be asked for nursing advice in grocery stores, in family circles, in neighborhoods, while traveling, and even when you are on vacation. How you respond to these individuals will be as important as how you care for your patient in a hospital, clinic, or nursing home. Look upon your career in nursing as an adventure and learn to be open and ready for the unexpected. As a nurse, your life is open to so many avenues and roads. Where you choose to go and what you choose to do have endless possibilities. Never say 'no' and never give up because the rewards are priceless on this earth and in heaven. God bless you in your journey!"

Sister Victoria Marie Indyk, PhD

Associate Professor of Nursing
Madonna University
College of Nursing and Health
Livonia, MI

Expertise:
Medical - Surgical Nursing - 10 years
St. Mary Mercy Hospital, Livonia, MI
Geriatric Nursing - 8 years - Director of Nursing
Felician Sisters Infirmary, Livonia, MI
Nursing Supervisor - 4 years
St. Francis Nursing Home, Saginaw, MI
Nurse Educator - 13 years
Madonna University, College of Nursing, Livonia, MI

Education:
Madonna University (BSN, MSN)
Wayne State University (PhD in Nursing)

66 A 'B' and mental health is better than an 'A' and insanity."

"Forgiveness is easier to get than permission."

"Salt and Stress = >> Systolic BP."

SHERI INNERARITY, RN, PhD, FNP, ACNS
Associate Professor for Clinical Nursing
The University of Texas at Austin
Austin, TX
Expertise:
Teaching
Adult Clinical Nurse Specialist
Family Nurse Practitioner
Education:
University of Texas at Austin (FNP)
Texas Women's University (PhD)
University of Texas at Austin (MSN,BSN)
Midwestern University (ADN)

((There is so much a seasoned nurse can tell you about how to be a better nurse and how to build your career.

I have found that when you live your life well, other important things fall into place. Part of living your life well means taking very good care of yourself. Nurses tend to be givers, constantly taking care of others (patients, families, spouses, friends). You must practice and learn to take care of yourself. This is excellent role modeling for your patients, children and everyone you come into contact with. In addition, it helps to set clear boundaries with others. Taking care of yourself helps in preventing burn out. The people you care for need you to take care of yourself so you don't allow yourself to grow sick and tired and unable to do the job of healing.

Second, have fun! Find ways to make your work enjoyable. Challenge and stretch yourself and watch yourself grow in amazing ways. Good luck to all of you in your nursing careers and in your lives. Nursing is one of the most meaningful careers and I hope you all find it as rewarding as I have."

Sarah L. Katula, APRN, BC, PhD

Professor
Elmhurst College
Clinical Nurse Specialist
Advocate Good Samaritan Hospital in Illinois
Elmhurst, IL

Expertise:
Psychiatric Clinical Nurse Specialist
Domestic Violence Research and Community Work

Education:
Valparaiso University
Rush University (Masters)
UIC (Ph.D.)

❝ See the sacred in every person."

"Develop your listening skills; a skilled listener makes for a skilled clinician."

"Always leave the patient with a positive feedback and a smile."

GREGORY P. KNAPIK, DNP, PHD
Assistant Professor of Nursing
University of Akron
Akron, OH
Expertise:
Primary Healthcare and Wellness,
Especially to the Marginalized and Uninsured
Education:
Joint PhD in Nursing Program
Kent State University/University of Akron
Case Western Reserve University

“ Honor your patients enough to do what needs to be done.”

"Many students and new nurses are hesitant to 'enter a patient's personal space' or to provide 'physical care' to patients for a variety of reasons: limited exposure, fear of hurting someone or making someone uncomfortable, etc. When a student or new nurse embraces this concept of 'honoring' the patient, the novice becomes more comfortable in performing both basic and more complex nursing interventions."

JUDY KREIDEWEIS, MSN, RN
Assistant Professor of Nursing
Northwestern State University of Louisiana
Natchitoches, LA
Extended campus: Alexandria, LA
Expertise:
Medical-Surgical Nursing
Nursing Education
Education:
St. Joseph Hospital School of Nursing
Northwestern State University of Louisiana (MSN)

❝ Through all the physical and emotional hard work, and it is hard work indeed, remember that it is a privilege and honor to be with patients at some of the most significant times in their lives: birth, death, joy and sorrow."

JUDITH LAMBTON, MS, RN, EdD
Professor
University of San Francisco
San Francisco, CA
Expertise:
Critical Care
Pediatrics
Education:
Presbyterian-St Luke
University of California at San Francisco

“ Work hard. Nothing comes easy. Set your goals and strive to reach them.”

“Always think positive and in terms of success.”

Kari R. Lane, MSN, RN
Assistant Professor
South Dakota State University
Brookings, SD
Expertise:
Cardiac Critical Care
Emergency
Public Health
Education:
Iowa Methodist School of Nursing (RN)
Drake University College of Nursing (BSN, MSN)

❝ Having just celebrated my 35th year in professional nursing, I can say without reservation that I have never regretted my decision to become a nurse. My practice has spanned populations ranging from micropremies to centenarians, my oldest patient in wound care having attained the ripe old age of 104 years young. I have worked in hospitals, clinics, nursing schools, and private practice with roles as diverse as staff nurse to chief nursing officer and simulation instructor to associate dean. I have been happy more than sad, fulfilled more than frustrated. I have welcomed human beings into the world and held their hands and cried with their families as they left the world behind. I have never been bored. In summing up my wisdom to offer the next generation of nurses, this is what I would say by way of a mnemonic:

R: Risk getting to know your patients; really involve yourself in the affective domain.

E: Energize your practice; have a PASSION for what you do.

G: Grow: never stop reading, studying, changing.

I: Involve yourself in policy or others will decide what is best for your profession.

S: Smile often, laugh loud and have a good time; endorphins are wonderful.

T: Transform bedside care through the use of best evidence. Never say, 'But we've always done it this way.'

E: Express your ideas; challenge others; collaborate.

R: React quickly and rationally to emergencies; don't wait for others to act first.

E: Engage your critics; you can learn from all points of view.

D: Demand the best from yourself and your colleagues. The highest level of achievement never comes from accepting the status quo.

N: Nurture all those around you including yourself. You can't care for others unless you take care of yourself.

U: Understand that nothing worth doing is easy. Nursing will give you the best and worst days of your life. You'll learn something from each experience.

R: Respect all your co-workers from housekeeping through the top levels of administration. You may be the quarterback of patient care but you need all those linemen to help you move the ball across the goal line.

S: Synergy results when two or more individuals work together to achieve something better than what can be accomplished individually. The whole is always greater than the sum of its parts.

E: Empower those around you. As Yoda said, 'Do or do not. There is no try.'"

Karen C. Lyon, PhD, APRN, ACNS

Associate Dean & Professor
Nelda C. Stark College of Nursing
Texas Woman's University
Houston, TX

Expertise:
Wound Care and Hyperbaric Medicine
Servant Leadership
Professional Role Development
Competency Outcomes

Education:
University of Texas System School of Nursing (BSN)
University of Texas at El Paso (MSN)

Courage: Have the courage to question health care providers when an order does not seem appropriate for the patient. You'll learn the rationale for the order and perhaps 'catch an error.'"

"Errors: Learn from errors—every nurse will make at least one or more errors at some time in his/her career. Protect the patient by reporting the error, think about why the error occurred and change the behavior that caused the error."

"Medications: NEVER give a medication with which you are not familiar—that places the patient in harm's way."

"Busy: Your days will always be extremely busy-that is the nature of the profession that you have chosen. Do not whine—it is irritating, unattractive and does not solve anything. Get involved with task forces and committees to change nursing practice instead of just complaining."

"Love your profession: When mediocre care becomes 'good enough' it is time to leave nursing! Your patients deserve more than mediocre and so do you."

BERNADETTE MADARA, EdD, BC, APRN
Professor – Nursing
Southern Connecticut State University
New Haven, CT
Expertise:
Adult Health
Education:
St. Anselm College (BSN)

❝ Never say it is the Q-word (quiet), because you will be sorry!"

"Every day is a gift."

"It is amazing to me to see some of the toughest guys cry when their mothers (whom they have shunned) are the only ones who visit them."

"Every day spent in the hospital increases the patient's chance of harm."

"Surround yourself with folks you would want to care for you."

"Never work in a unit (place) where you wouldn't want to be a patient."

"Remember that most trauma patients would have ended up in someone's ICU; they just happened to end up in yours."

"We are all human and we need to learn from our mistakes and figure out what we can do to prevent them from happening within our walls."

"That could have been me."

"Treat your patient as you would want to be treated because one day you may be in that bed."

"What would Florence do?"

"When dealing with surveyors remember they are trying to keep you safe from yourself."

"When it comes to surveyors you don't have to be right, you just have to be successful."

"Remember that your patients know themselves a whole lot better than you do."

"Work-arounds are only as good as the nurse who remembers what they are."

"One nurse, one patient, one day."

JULI MAXWORTHY, DNP, MSN, MBA, RN, CNL, CPHQ
Senior Director, Quality & Care Management
Saint Francis Memorial Hospital
Part Time Faculty, University of San Francisco
CEO, WithMax Consulting
San Francisco, CA

Expertise:
Critical Care
Quality, Performance Improvement
Risk, Case Management

Education:
California State University, Hayward (RN)
Holy Names University (MSN/MBA)
University of San Francisco (DNP)

" Listen to your patient; it will save your butt every time!!"

"There's a method to the madness…. Read the label, read the label, read the label."

"I am so much more afraid of the student or nurse that doesn't ask questions."

TONJA MCCLAIN, MS, RN
Faculty
Ball State University School of Nursing
Muncie, IN
Expertise:
Obstetrics
Community Health
Education:
University of Kentucky (BSN)
Ball State University (MSN)

On fatal diagnosis:
"There are worse things than death."

On what patients pray for:
"Acceptance of what is doesn't negate what could be."

MARY O'CONNOR, PhD, RN
Assistant Clinical Professor of Nursing
University of Missouri Kansas City
Kansas City, MO
Expertise:
Perinatal Care
Education:
St. Louis University

" When taking care of pediatric patients, silence is not golden."

"If the patient is yelling: They have an airway; They are protecting their airway."

"All bleeding stops . . . eventually. When it stops may be up to you."

"If you think about doing it, do it."

Margaret O'Donnell, BSN, EMT-P, CEN, CMTE
Program Manager
UNC Carolina Air Care: Critical Care Transport
Chapel Hill, NC
Expertise:
Emergency Nursing
Critical Care Transport, Air and Ground
Education:
Crouse Irving Memorial Hospital School of Nursing
Syracuse, New York

"STAY IN SCHOOL. If you wish to be taken seriously by other members of the health care team, like physicians, pharmacists, nutritionists, physical therapists, speech therapists, and others, you need to have more than an associate or diploma degree. Earning a degree in a community college is a great beginning but it should not be the end of your nursing education. You owe it to yourself, to your patients and to your profession to pursue higher levels of nursing education. Pursuing a higher degree in nursing also gives you the opportunity to give something back to the profession and to make a contribution beyond just that of your individual patient assignments. It's a shame that 80% of associate degree and baccalaureate nursing graduates never pursue a higher level degree. When I returned to school to earn a masters degree in critical care and trauma nursing I was shocked at how much this higher level learning process improved my nursing care and how much it expanded my ability to think in even non-nursing areas of my life. Earning a PhD in nursing was a deconstructing-reconstructing process that was both existential and spiritual; a lasting human growth experience. Today, I can't imagine what life would be like without having gone through the process of earning graduate degrees."

Liana Orsolini-Hain, PhD, RN, CCRN

Nursing Instructor
City College of San Francisco
Committee Member
Institute of Medicine & Robert Wood Johnson Fndn
Initiative on the Future of Nursing
San Francisco, CA

Expertise:
Nursing Education
Workforce Development
Medical Surgical Nursing
Critical Care and Emergency Room Nursing

Education:
University of California, San Francisco

On the patient:

"Before each patient encounter center yourself and leave any distractions at the door. Focus only on the patient and the patient's family. Treat each patient as if they were a beloved member of your family. Do not be judgmental. Remember the centrality of the patient and know that you have the power to create either a negative or positive healing milieu with your words and actions. At the end of the day ensure that you have done your very best for your patient because you were truly present for every patient encounter."

On the nurse:

"There is no profession that compares to nursing. Nurses have the distinct honor and privilege of caring for individuals at their most vulnerable times. This allows the nurse the opportunity to live life at a very deep level. Nurses share the most precious human life experiences of birth and death; caring for others through their pain and joy; from illness to wellness. Nurses are given an opportunity for transcendence in life through these moments of caring for others. As we engage in this work of nursing, these moments are magnificent and awe-inspiring. However, never forget that your first duty is to yourself; If you do not care for yourself, you cannot care effectively for others."

On the environment:

"There is no question that nurses render care in a chaotic, fast-paced healthcare delivery system. Be always cognizant of your impact on this environment. We know that the environment can either heal or harm our patients. It can also be toxic to us. The stress that surrounds nurses creates a place for potential negative energy that must be counterbalanced by appropriate responses to that negativity. Disruptive behavior among healthcare professionals is an unfortunate reality. To help counterbalance this, never forget the centrality of the patient. Remember that we must work together to create an environment that is healing not only to the patients we care for, but to ourselves as well."

BRENDA PETERSEN, MSN, RN, CPNP, CNL
Faculty Associate
Seton Hall University College of Nursing
South Orange, NJ
Expertise:
Nationally Certified Pediatric Nurse Practitioner and
Clinical Nurse Leader
Pediatric Nursing in Primary Care, Acute Care, and
Community Health.
Education:
Seton Hall University

❝ In the decade I have been teaching undergraduate nursing students I have gathered a litany of truisms that I have designated 'Peterson's Platitudes.' I deliver my account of the facts with authority and passion, giving the students the impression I am imparting something of great value. I tell my students that nursing demands a robust knowledge base, skilled clinical reasoning and judgment, proficient skills and above all, a sense of humor. A nurse with a sense of humor can and will survive the most [insert adjective here, i.e., embarrassing, anxiety-provoking, sad, rage-producing, heartrending] event and continue to provide care to the best of their ability in trying times. Live your profession with passion or do something else!

Nursing attire:

- If you are wearing something white at the beginning of the shift, it will not be white at the end of the shift.
- If you are using betadine for anything, some of it will permanently stain your favorite scrubs.
- Your uniform shouldn't double as an outfit for an exotic dancer.
- No woman looks good in a hair cover, goggles, face shield/mask, and gown unless she is wearing dramatic eye make-up.
- Pre-, peri-, and post-menopausal nurses are not

meant to wear plastic gowns, even for short periods of time.

Standard precautions:

- Blood, vomit, and feces are NOT fashion accessories.
- A patient ALWAYS vomits more than the emesis basin holds.
- A patient ALWAYS vomits on the clean linen, not the dirty linen, when you are changing the bed.
- The number of times a patient soils the bed during your shift is directly proportional to the number of wash clothes missing from the linen cart.
- When in doubt, wash your hands.

Tips of the trade:

- The sharp end of anything ALWAYS goes toward the patient.
- If the patient is over 75 years of age and doesn't respond to verbal or physical stimuli, they are either deaf or dead.
- You can't fix dead, nor can you make it worse. So, calm down!
- There will be patients you don't like, relate to, respect, etc. Carry those feelings in your heart, not on your face.
- If the patient tells you, 'I feel like I am going to die,' believe him, no matter what the monitor says.
- If you are going to fail, fail BIG and do it with PASSION. You won't make that same mistake again.
- Your first Foley insertion on a live patient will

be on a confused, agitated, combative, severely overweight female. Be mindful of aseptic technique.

- Don't forget to unplug the code cart on the way to the patient's room. A flying defibrillator doesn't hasten the patient's recovery.
- 'See one, do one' is NOT a successful teaching/learning strategy.
- Patients live in spite of what we do to them.
- The art of nursing is establishing a relationship of trust in less than 15 minutes before you have to touch the patient intimately.
- The base of power should rest firmly with the patient, not the nurse.
- If the patient is circling the drain, you have no IV access.
- If the patient is talking and making sense, the patient is hemodynamically stable.
- When a patient asks, 'Have you done this before?' he doesn't have to know it was on a mannequin in the lab. Say, 'yes' with confidence.

Time management:

- The minute you have your day organized with a fool-proof plan of attack, one of your patients will start circling the drain.
- The minute you have your day organized with a fool-proof plan of attack, the charge nurse will change your assignment.
- Floating to another unit has many similarities to waking up in a foreign country where you don't speak the language.
- The number of call-ins is directly proportional to the number of patients in your assignment.

- Divide your assignment into three categories: 1) things I must do, 2) things I would like to do, and 3) 'if this were a perfect world' I would accomplish this, too."

Cynthia Peterson, MS, RN
Assistant Professor
Department of Nursing
Husson University
Bangor, ME
Expertise:
Medical Surgical Nursing
Critical Care Nursing
Clinical Simulation
Education:
Husson University (BSN)
Arizona State University (MS)

** ❝** Inspirational Message to Aspiring Nurses:

Most of us in the nursing profession find that we go through life in the fast lane. It is a hectic pace with responsibilities of work, family and often school or continuing education always competing for what is the priority for the moment. If we want to be the best nurses that we can be, we need to stay on top of the constant influx of new technology, knowledge, competencies and ever-emerging ways to improve the work that we do. The nursing profession carries with it many demands and along with those demands come many rewards.

At the end of a busy day, we leave with a mind full of what we have done to make life better for others. We hope and pray that we have covered all the bases, hung all the IV's, administered all the meds and taken the time to provide the empathy, care and warmth that accompanies our responsibilities for care. While we were busy for the day, we take away a strong sense of gratification in helping others in so many ways. Our love of caring for people brought us to accept this profession as our own. Our love of caring for people sustains us even in the most difficult times. This is the essence of what it means to be a nurse.

I have had the joy of being a nurse for the last 42 years with many years of experience in staff nursing along with being a nurse educator. As a professor at a local community college, I am moved by the men and women who aspire to be nurses. Throughout the rigorous program of study to become a nurse, individuals eagerly put forth effort to be sure to gain the knowledge and skills necessary to become the best nurses that they can be. The caring component simply falls into place. However, caring is essential and most of the time, the aspiring student knows this without a measure of a doubt. Most enter nursing because they want to work with people and help people.

As I have gone through my career, I have never for a moment thought that I should have chosen another profession. Nursing has provided rewards that have been multi-dimensional. From these rewards, one gains the sense of self actualization in the work that they accomplish. It is a major commitment to be a nurse and one that carries with it the joys and sorrows of life. It is most rewarding and my own advice for anyone considering this profession is to follow your inner self. If there is a calling for you to be a nurse, it will be heard."

THERESA L. PIEKUT, MSN
Professor of Nursing
Community College of Allegheny County
Pittsburgh, PA
Expertise:
Nursing Education
Maternal-Newborn Nursing
Education:
University of Pittsburgh

**   ** While caring is not enough, when you no longer care, it is time to do something different."

"Nursing is a 24/7 role of privilege with commensurate responsibility."

"Be the nurse you will need when you need help; set an example."

"Appreciate the honor of caring for others and bearing witness to life's most intimate and challenging moments."

"If the bureaucracy is burdensome, work to change it. Don't walk away complaining."

"Nurse with no regrets. Your patients deserve nothing less."

E. Carol Polifroni, EdD, CNE, NEA-BC, RN

Associate Professor
University of Connecticut School of Nursing
Storrs, CT

Expertise:
39 Years of Nursing:
Staff Nurse
Administration
In-service Education
Education of Pre-licensure and Post-licensure Students
Academic Administration
Research
Writing
Consulting

Education:
Saint Anselm College

❝ Nursing is a wonderful profession with multiple opportunities waiting to be seized. Nurses should remain mission-driven with a vision for their own personal growth and development while utilizing this energy to impact their patients, families, communities and society. Success is dependent upon personal self-awareness, nursing knowledge, experience, and social networks. The key to maintaining success is securing life-long mentoring and remaining actively engaged as a citizen of the nursing profession. Knowledge attainment is a continuous process. Know thyself and utilize your assets and continually improve your weaknesses. Life is a journey, changes is inevitable and constant. Your success is dependent on the road chosen for this journey and your response to change."

Demetrius J. Porche, DNS, PhD, APRN, FAANP, FAAN

Dean and Professor
Louisiana State University Health Sciences Center –
School of Nursing
New Orleans, LA

Expertise:
Men's Health
Leadership
Publishing
Primary Care
Nursing Education

Education:
Nicholls State University
Louisiana State University Medical Center

❝ A simple 'thank you' from a child after a procedure can make even the darkest day seem bright!"

"You just never know what 'treasures' a pediatric patient is hiding in which orifice, or why!"

"The sickest pediatric patients have better dispositions than most of the well population."

KATHY PROWS, RN, MSN, FNP
Adjunct Clinical Faculty
USF School of Nursing
San Francisco, CA
Expertise:
Pediatric
Education:
University of San Francisco

On Teaching Nursing Students:

"Teach your students to the standard you want the nurse caring for your family member to maintain."

"The nurse who does everything she is supposed to do and does it correctly is the average nurse. The student who does everything she is supposed to do and does it correctly, is an average student and earns a grade of 'C.' If you want to earn an 'A,' show me the evidence that your work is more than just correct!"

"Learning, like nursing, requires presence. If you are not present, you will miss the opportunity forever. Patients do not wait to give birth until it is convenient for the nurse. You need to be present."

"Remember the curriculum was created for a purpose: to educate nurses. When a course ends, you need to carry the knowledge of the course forward as it is the foundation of all the courses that follow."

On Perinatal or Maternal/Infant Nursing:

"One of the most complex patients is the newborn infant. There is no existing medical record, everything is brand new and untested, and they cannot tell us if something is wrong."

"Perinatal nurses not only help bring babies into the world, but help to begin new families."

"A father of a baby in the NICU once said, 'I thought it would be like taking my car to the garage – a quart of oil, a gallon of gas and all is well. Then I watched the nurses and learned it is so much more complex and they have so much knowledge.'"

"When caring for sick children remember the way of *HELP*:
- H: humanize the environment
- E: eliminate separation from the family
- L: life routines familiar to the child
- P: preparation – for procedures, for the family, for the known and the unknown."

"The textbook states that the complication rate is less than 1%, but if it happens to your patient it is 100%."

On Being a Post-Partum Nurse:

"The uterus shrinks, the perineum aches, the breast gives milk. The baby is trusting, the mother is learning, the family has grown; Who are they, what will they become; change, adaptation and growth; The post-partum experience - share it, cherish it."

On Supervising Students in the Clinical Setting

"When I approach a student a couple of hours into the clinical experience and they say, 'I have finished everything except the patient assessment,' I ask, 'How can you do *anything* without the assessment?'"

Deborah A. Raines, PhD, RN, ANEF
Director of the Scholarship of Teaching
Professor
Florida Atlantic University
Boca Raton, FL
Expertise:
Perinatal Nursing
Obstetrical and Neonatal Care
Nursing Education
Education:
Syracuse University (BSN)
University of Pennsylvania (MSN)
Virginia Commonwealth University:
Medical College of Virginia (PhD)

" It is likely that about half of the 'evidence' in healthcare is in reality true. We just don't know which half!"

"People don't care about how much you know until they know how much you care!"

"One key to success is to do the common thing uncommonly well."

Luann Richardson, CRNP, PhD
Assistant Professor
Duquesne University
Pittsburgh, PA
Expertise:
Evidence-Based Practice Instruction
Education:
University of Pittsburgh

" Assessing your patient without the technology: So much is learned by the 'Eyeball Test,' which simply stated means, 'Does your patient look good or does your patient look bad?'"

Diane Rudolphi, RN, MS
Clinical Instructor
University of Delaware
Newark, DE
Expertise:
Medical Surgical Nursing Instructor
Education:
Texas Christian University (BSN)
University of Maryland (MS)

" We have been monitoring the air and water for the presence of toxic chemicals for a long time. In the last decade we have begun to monitor human blood and urine, and even breast milk, for the presence of toxic chemicals that should never be in our bodies. The results of these 'biomonitoring' efforts are alarming. We have found that hundreds of toxic chemicals are now circulating in our bodies. With them comes a wide array of health risks – cancer, infertility, developmental delays, neurodegenerative diseases and more. Even umbilical cord blood – blood that is circulating in a newborn's body at the time of birth – is now awash in solvents, pesticides, plasticizers and other potentially toxic chemicals. In 2010, the American Nurses Association established an environmental health standard of practice for the profession of nursing, meaning that environmental health is now a requisite component of our profession. As such, it is critical that we understand the contribution that environmental toxicants play in the overall disease burden in our population. All nurses now have a professional obligation to learn about the relationship between our environment and human health effects. It is important for us to assess our patients and the communities we serve for the types of environmental exposures they may have. Just as we ask patients about their smoking and drinking habits, we should ask them about their work exposures and potentially harmful behaviors like the use of pesticides in their homes. We can encourage them to eat food that has been grown in a healthier manner thus reducing the use of pesticides, growth hormones, and unnecessary antibiotics.

In our own workplaces (hospitals, schools, clinics), nurses are taking the lead in 'greening' health care. We have been eliminating mercury-containing thermometers and other health care equipment; influencing our purchasing practices to buy environmentally-preferable products that are healthier for patients, employees, and the environment; and engaging in activities to better manage health care waste. There is much for nurses to learn about in this emerging and critical area of human health and many new roles for us to play. We can easily incorporate environmental risks into our assessments and patient/community education efforts. We also can use our voices in the policy arena to advocate for environmentally sound policies that protect human health. This is a critical time for the earth and its people, and nurses are the right people at this critical time to be engaged in making positive changes."

Barbara Sattler, RN, DrPH, FAAN

Professor
University of Maryland School of Nursing
Baltimore, MD

Expertise:

Environmental Health

- Work in the fields of occupational and environmental health for more than 30 years with experience in the non-profit/advocacy world, labor, and currently in an academic position for 20 years.

- Director of the Environmental Health Education Center at the University of Maryland which has the only graduate program for nurses that focuses explicitly on environmental health. The Center has been a regional lead training center, responsible for community outreach under an EPA Hazardous Substance Research Center grant, hosted a model state program for engaging the health care sector in sustainability efforts, and supported a NIEHS community-based, environmental justice research project.

- Service on IOM committees on environmental health information, on the Maryland State Environmental Justice Commission, and the Children's Health Protection Policy Advisory Committee to the US EPA.

- Helped to found the Alliance of Nurses for Healthy Environments, a national consortium of individual nurses and nursing organizations which is addressing education, practice, research, and policy/advocacy issues.

- Registered Nurse with a Masters and Doctoral Degree from the Johns Hopkins School of Public Health.

Education:

Pilgrim State Hospital School of Nursing
John Hopkins School of Public Health

❝ When an experienced nurse is concerned about a patient, pay attention; knowledge and intuition are powerful devices."

"You'll know when you are a nurse when patient advocacy is a passion."

LAURA K. SCHENK, PHD, RN, NNP-BC
Associate Professor
School of Nursing
University of Mississippi Medical Center
Jackson, MS
Expertise:
Pediatrics
Neonatal
Education:
College of St. Theresa (BS)
School of Nursing
University of Mississippi Medical Center, (MSN)
University of Mississippi Medical Center, (PhD)

" In my long career encompassing being a nurse, nurse academician and academic leader, in general, I have found that we as nurses are 'long' on being pragmatic and capable - but 'not as long' on taking the lead to forge new models or create 'disruptive innovations.' We work hard to make things happen but often while standing behind others in the lead - perhaps less visible as to contribution.

Show your leadership colors! For stepping up and leading (creating, designing and testing) novel change, I recommend the following reminder or self-talk:

It's not a risk if there is no 'fear of failure', it's merely a trial! During a trial, there is always the potential to 'course correct' if or when implementation proves that the plan was insufficient or new opportunities emerge.

I believe that we do well to initiate a change element as a 'beginning,' meant to evolve continuously, mostly with no planned end. To be enamored with planning that is too lengthy, detailed and complete runs the risk of being 'stuck in planning,' shortchanging the potential, or en route failing to see options that would grow the capacity or excellence of the initiative."

JOAN L. SHAVER, PhD, RN, FAAN
Professor and Dean
University of Arizona College of Nursing
Tucson, AZ

Expertise:
Women's Health
Sleep Science

Education:
University of Alberta (Canada)
University of Washington (Seattle)

" In this era of advanced technology, do not forget the art of nursing. Florence Nightingale had the right idea - keep the patient clean, offer proper food and fresh air, wash your hands, stop and listen."

"Stay humble; the patient trusts you with his/her life and no one is above making a mistake so forgive yourself and move on."

PAULA SICILIANO, DNP, APRN, GNP-C
Director of the Nurse Practitioner Program
Associate Professor
Nurse Practitioner in Internal Medicine
University of Utah College of Nursing
Midvale, UT
Expertise:
Geriatric Medicine
Education:
University of Utah

Being the best does not mean you will be the most liked, but you will be respected."

"Do not determine your value based on the opinions of others, but rather base your value by recognizing who God created you to be."

"In order to safely arrive at the end of your journey, you may have to dispose of excessive baggage."

"Some relationships are in your life for just a season, but problems arise when you try to hold onto them for a lifetime."

E'LORIA SIMON-CAMPBELL, RN, MSN, PHD(C)
Clinical Assistant Professor
Prairie View A & M University College of Nursing
Houston, TX
Expertise:
Nursing Education
Medical/Surgical Nursing
Online Education
Health Disparities: Hypertension in African Americans
Education:
University of Texas at Tyler (MSN 2005) (PhD May 2011)
Prairie View A&M University (BS Nursing 1995)

On testifying in court:

"Every professional opinion must be based on scientific evidence or evidence-based practices. Personal opinion has no place in a court room."

On death investigation:

"The deceased client is telling you what happened…look, listen, and feel to find all of the clues. They are right in front of you."

On examining a child:

"No one should ever hold a child down for an exam, especially a sexual assault exam. Doing this makes you no better than the perpetrator that assaulted the child."

On pediatric care:

"Just because a child is breathing, it doesn't mean he's breathing adequately. Listen to his chest-that's why you have that thing [stethoscope] around your neck."

On patient care:

"When in doubt, shout out! Ask for help and use your resources. Nursing is a team sport and there is no 'I' in team!"

"If your senses tell you something isn't right, believe it! Something isn't right!!!"

On lab values and other diagnostic tests:

"An excellent diagnostician relies on a thorough assessment, rather than waiting on a bunch of numbers from lab tests or arterial blood gases. These tests only reinforce what you have already diagnosed."

On triage:

"From across the room, many triage nurses are able to accurately determine the severity of one's illness. Just use your senses-look and listen."

On dying:

"If a patient tells you they feel like they are going to die, believe them. They will die in a relatively short time after telling this to you."

DEBORAH L. ST. GERMAIN, DNP, RN, CEN
Assistant Professor of Clinical Nursing
New Orleans, LA
Expertise:
Forensic Nursing
Emergency Nursing
Critical Care Nursing
Education:
University of Tennessee Health Science Center (DNP)
Louisiana State University Health Sciences Center (MN)
Murray State University (BSN)

66 Throughout your nursing career, approach each new day with passion, cherish relationships, make reflection a daily habit, and accumulate the positive stories in your sacred bundle."

KAREN STEFANIAK, RN, PHD
Assistant Professor
University of Kentucky College of Nursing
Lexington, KY
Expertise:
Administration
Education:
Lakeview Memorial Hospital School of Nursing (Diploma)
Southern Illinois University (BSN)
University of Kentucky (MSN, PhD)

“ My philosophy to self and nursing students:

The 3 L's:

Love　　　　Love yourself so you can love others.

Learning　　Learn all that you can; it will help you to grow as you continue to live, work (and love).

Laughter　　Don't forget to laugh; it will help everyone and everything around you everyday.”

JEANNE VENHAUS STEIN, RN, MSN
Assistant Professor of Nursing
California State University at Long Beach
Long Beach, CA
Expertise:
Psychiatric Mental Nursing
Clinical Nurse Specialist in Community Mental Health
Nurse Educator
Nurse Humorist
Education:
University of Colorado Denver Health Science Center

" Look after yourself in order to remain passionate about nursing, insist on high standards, and be ready to give of yourself because we nurses do make a difference in other's lives."

JANE SUMNER, PhD, RN, APRN, BC
Professor of Nursing
School of Nursing
Louisiana State University Health Science Center
New Orleans, LA
Expertise:
Theorist in Caring in Nursing
Advanced Public Health
Community Health Nursing Instruction
Education:
Hutt Hospital School of Nursing
Lower Hutt, New Zealand (RN)
BSN, MN, PhD all in the US

((Every experience with a client will add to or decrease your spiritual core. Guard your compassion, exercise your tolerance, risk living that opportunity."

ANNE TROY, RN, MN, FNP
Assistant Professor of Nursing
Louisiana State University Health Sciences Center
School of Nursing
New Orleans, LA
Expertise:
Mental Health
Forensics
Education:
Rutgers University

“ Turning your back on a student can be like turning your back on the ocean.”

MARY PAT ULICNY, RN, MS
Clinical Instructor
Clinical Simulation Lab Coordinator
University of Maryland School of Nursing
Baltimore, MD
Expertise:
Clinical Simulation
Clinical Instructor Adult Medical Surgical Nursing
Adult Critical Care
Education:
Duquesne University School of Nursing

❝ I have devoted my career to the education of nursing students, the primary care needs of the elderly and their caregivers, and issues associated with the aging of the RN workforce. I have been an advocate of elders when it was not popular and when it was popular but I have always known that elders do not have enough advocates and devoted my career to training nurses who will follow in my footsteps and provide safe, optimal care to this vulnerable population. Working with elders is rewarding and heartbreaking but we must all understand that in too short a time, 'we' will become 'them.'

On dealing with elders:

"The minute a doctor enters the room, the nurse ceases to exist."

"The elder will do anything that a doctor asks them to do, no matter how difficult they have been to the nursing staff."

"The elder will tell the nurse everything but does not want to bother the doctor, as he is so busy."

"In the absence of a doctor, a male nurse can enter the elder's room and the elder will automatically assume he is a doctor and do what is asked of him without argument."

"Elders are the most engaging, enlightening, rewarding, and maddening group of patients a nurse will ever have."

On patient autonomy:

"Never assume because one is elderly that they should have limited autonomy. We would hate this and so do they."

On interacting with elderly patients:

"Never speak to a family member first, look at them when asking the elder questions, or assume that the elder needs someone to speak for them. Once you treat the elder this way they no longer trust you."

On interacting with caregivers of the elderly:

"Never assume that the caregiver has the elder's best interests at heart, this may not be the case."

"Be alert for signs of abuse of any elder under your care. Remember, abuse, like incest, begins at home."

On caring for nursing home patients:

"Always remember that this is their HOME, not a hospital and never, never, never refer to this type of facility as 'God's Waiting Room.'"

"Make sure that you understand that the two greatest privileges we can have as nurses is to be with someone when they draw their first breath and when they draw their last breath."

"Treat every patient and family as if they were yours."

JOYCE MCCULLERS VARNER,
DNP, GNP-BC, GCNS
Clinical Associate Professor
University of South Alabama College of Nursing
Mobile, AL
Expertise:
Geriatrics
Caregiving
Dementia Care
Nursing Education
Research Interests: Dementia, Family Caregiving Issues,
Palliative Care Needs
Education:
University of South Alabama

“ I teach a class in the School of Nursing entitled, 'History of Nursing.' In our class in the fall 2009 semester, I had our students pretend that they were actually nursing alongside Florence Nightingale. They were to pretend that they were involved in helping the soldiers injured in the Crimean War and were to write a letter to someone about their experiences. The letter below was the one I composed in a character like Florence Nightingale. This letter represents my major words of wisdom for nurses. Nurses should always learn from those who have come before them. We must remember that we stand on the shoulders of all nurses, throughout history and in our personal lives, who have given us valuable lessons which are ageless.

November 1854

Dearest Sister,

I find this month the most trying and heart weary of my life. Oh, Sister, how my bones and muscles hurt, but what is most troubling is the pain in my heart and soul. I have always known that God was my guiding light and the sun that brought light to the darkest side of man. I believe that God had a mission for my life. However, in the quiet and darkness of this moonless night, I find myself questioning all my beliefs.

On my way to Scutari, how my heart soared. I was planning all the things that needed to be organized and done to help the brave young men of our Queen's military. What a privileged and sacred trust had been given to me and the fine young women who have followed me to this hallowed ground. As I contemplated on all the work that needed to be done, I prayed to God that I had the intellect and strength to implement the things I had learned at Kaiserwerth with my dear friends and mentors, Theodor and Frederike. Sister, I am so fearful that I will fail at this grand undertaking. So much depends upon the work we do in this most wretched place. I had hoped that our work here would provide proof of the principles of nursing as I learned them at Kaiserwerth. There must be a time and place to prove the value of God's work through the minds, hearts, and hands of these new nurses. Now I wonder at the arrogance of my grandiose belief that I could change the view of all these men who are in control of everything at Scutari. They do not want us here and hamper our efforts at every turn. Why, why dearest Sister, should anyone harbor ill will towards my brave young nurses who only want to help alleviate the pain and suffering of the wounded and dying? How such pettiness can live in the hearts of those who say they care for the lives entrusted to them, I do not know.

The days start early and are so long; sixteen hour days of hearing the cries and prayers, and witnessing the suffering in the lives of such young men. These men, who should be with their wives and children playing in the fields, dancing at parties, or having drinks with their brothers, are hurt and dying. Their agony is beyond all words. Their screams fill my waking days and haunt my dreams. How God can let this happen and how we, a handful of nurses, can help is a mystery to me.

When we arrived at the hospital, I felt there had been a mistake, for surely this long tin building could not provide shelter, much less the environment for healing. My nurses and I had brought what supplies we could carry in the wagons. No one would help us unload the supplies. This was our first introduction to the disdain that the military officers and physicians held in their hearts and, by their actions, communicated to us.

As we were walking towards the entrance, the cold rain was falling in the fog and the thought crossed my mind that God was crying. But, was He crying for what we would see, what we would endure, or both? As the chill of the rain and cold soaked into my skin and muscles, I began to shake. I still do not know if it was the cold or fear that evoked my muscles to convulse. My next sense that was assaulted was smell. The smell of human waste, blood, burning wood, and meat so assaulted my sensibilities that I feared I would faint. I so wanted to cover my nose with a handkerchief that Mama gave me scented with her perfume. However, I dare not give any sign of weakness for all our detractors are watching intently for any sign of what they would call the hysteria of womanhood. I knew my physical body could not take any further insults, but somehow my legs moved and I walked into the hospital. It was at that time that I knew I had marched into Hell. Oh, Sister, such misery and suffering I could not have imagined in my darkest nightmare. Young men barely older than our friend, James, were laying in bloody vomit on covered straw beds, which lay on the floor. Rats, maggots, and fleas were everywhere. It was as if the floor moved as the vermin formed the sea of moving horror.

The wounded had bandages that were dry and crusted with blood and dirt. As my brave nurses and I walked between the rows of beds, hands reached up to clasp our hands. Voices which still had the high pitch of youth called to us to help, asking us to touch them and to pray for them. It was as if some strength that I did not know I possessed entered my body. This strength could have only come from my Higher Power and it enveloped me in a light that warmed my body and soul. It was at that moment that I knew we small band of nurses could make a difference. No longer would a British hero give his life alone in this horror without a nurse's touch and prayers as he made the transition from this world to the light of God's embrace.

During our first week, we set about making the hospital and patients clean. My nurses, so strong and tireless, worked night and day scrubbing every floor, wall, and surface in the hospital. Since there were no facilities for washing bedding and clothing, we rented a house in town to use as a laundry. Everything that touched the patient, we scrubbed by hand until our hands were raw and swollen. There was no money to rent this house because my military and physician superiors did not see any value to cleanliness. How I wish I could send these men of science and logical thought to Kaiserwerth so they could learn the lessons of hygiene, nutrition, fresh air, and spiritual comfort. So dear Sister, I have been using my own money to pay the rent for the laundry and to buy clothing for the patients. When we arrived, most of the patients did not have shirts and the month that we have been here, we have provided over three thousand shirts to the patients.

Our next most pressing problem has been making sure the patients have sufficient food for their fragile bodies to heal. How anyone could believe that one meal a day consisting mostly of potatoes, corn mash, and maybe a little meat could provide the energy necessary for healing is beyond belief. My nurses and I have scavenged the town to find fresh vegetables, bread, meat, and milk for the nutrition of our patients. We have set up a kitchen and prepare all the meals ourselves. Since the patients' well-being is our main concern, we have limited ourselves to one meal a day. Sister, please do not think this is sacrifice. The sacrifice has been made by these our brothers who have given of their blood for our country. When I think back to the life of privilege you and I were born into, I see it with different eyes and now a different heart. I am not the same person who left home for Scutari one month ago.

I now know what man is capable of doing in the name of a just cause. I know what suffering and horror looks like, smells like, and feels like. I also now know what courage, strength, faith, and integrity look like. They are no longer abstract, philosophical writings in a pompous library. They have names and faces. The names and faces of our patients and for me, the names and faces of my nurses. We have made a difference here at Scutari. In the months we have been here, the death rate has decreased by 50% and I am sure that we will continue to make a difference in these brave, young soldiers' lives. God has truly led me to my destiny.

I have been keeping careful records documenting everything we have done to improve the conditions here and its effect upon patient fatality reports. I believe this information is essential in proving the value of standardized nursing training.

It is late at night and it is time for me to make my visits to the patients. As I stare at the flame from my writing lamp, I see the light of God which connects all of us as brothers and sisters. There is no separateness when we honor the light of God within each other. If we do this, perhaps this horror will end and never be recreated. Now, I must visit my boys.

This is where my faith and strength is called upon the most for I know that many of these young men will pass into God's hands tonight. All I can do is make sure that they are not alone and feel a comforting touch before they pass.

Dearest Sister, I must ask of you this most difficult promise. If I do not return from this war, please visit each of my nurses and tell them how much their strength and courage has inspired me. Also, please visit the nurses at Kaiserwerth and tell them that they taught me how to be a professional nurse and a good leader. Their lessons saved many lives. Sister, please tell Mama and Papa that I have always loved and honored them, but that a Higher Power led me to my destiny and that they should rejoice that my life had meaning, love, and passion.

Always,

Your loving Sister"

GLENDA C. WALKER, DSN, RN
Director, Richard and Lucille DeWitt School of Nursing
Stephen F. Austin State University
Nacogdoches, TX
Expertise:
Innovations in Nursing Education and Remediation
PTSD with a Particular Focus on Family Violence
Education:
Troy State University-(BSN)
University of Alabama in Birmingham (MSN)
University of Alabama in Birmingham (DSN)

❝ When washing your hands between patients, be mindful, wash away the experience with the last patient, your personal concerns, and enter clean and open to the experience of the next patient."

ANN MARIE LEE WALTON, RN, MPH, OCN, CHES
Clinical Nurse IV, Inpatient Hematology/Oncology
North Carolina Cancer Hospital
Chapel Hill, NC
Expertise:
Eight years oncology nursing experience
Education:
UNC School of Nursing

“ Don't forget what you already know.”

"Remember to answer questions that your patients don't know how to ask."

Bryan A. Weber, PhD, ARNP
Associate Professor
University of Florida
Gainesville, FL
Expertise:
Family Practice Dyadic Social Support
Education:
York College of PA (BS)
Case Western Reserve University (MSN, Ph.D.)

" Learn to laugh. If you do not have or develop a sense of humor, you will not survive. Treat each patient as if he/she were a family member. Work as a team member; you cannot be all to all at the same time. When you need help, ask for it. When you see a peer needing help, please offer it willingly. The purpose of our profession is to provide the best quality of care possible to our patients. Treat others with respect and you will be treated as such, this includes physicians, ancillary staff, your peers and most of all, your patients.

MARY F. WESSINGER, MN, BC
Part-time Clinical Faculty
University of South Carolina College of Nursing
Part-time Staff RN
Palmetto Health Baptist, OB-GYN
Columbia, SC

Expertise:
27 Years of Experience in Direct Patient Care
5 Years Full time at Midlands Technical College
1 Year at USC College of Nursing
9 Years as Part- time Clinical Faculty
Fundamental, Med-Surg, and OB Nursing Instruction
Certified Perinatal Nurse
American Nurses Credentialing Center

Education:
University of South Carolina College of Nursing (BSN, MN)

" Pain is what the patient says it is."

"When in doubt, pull it out."

"If a patient tells you he is dying, believe him."

"Crocks die, too."

"On dealing with 'the arrogant': 'So, were you born with universal knowledge?'"

"Tenderness precedes redness. Listen to the patient when he says something hurts."

"Regarding traumatic death: Allow significant others the option of viewing the deceased."

"Regarding miscarriage: Allow the mother to decide whether to view the remains. When something comes out of their body; most people want to look at it."

"When asked to perform something you aren't comfortable doing: 'No' is a complete sentence. But it helps to give your rationale."

"Never administer a drug if you don't know what it is used for."

"If a patient looks ill; they probably are. If a patient doesn't look ill, all bets are off."

"Prepare for the worst and it won't happen."

"If the staff is having a pot luck dinner, all hell breaking loose is a guarantee."

"Breast milk is human specific!"

"If you are burned out, rotate to OB/Newborn for six weeks."

"Never say that it's quiet on the unit. It won't be in five minutes if you use the 'Q- word.'"

CAROLYN MATHIS WHITE, JD, MSN, FNP-BC, PNP-BC
Clinical Professor
University of South Alabama College of Nursing
Fairhope, AL
Expertise:
Family and Pediatric Nursing
Education:
Polk Community College (Associate Degree 1979)
Auburn University (Bachelor of Science in Nursing 1993)
University of South Alabama (Masters of Science in Nursing 1996)

❝ One thing I know – as a GOOD Nurse:

A good nurse never takes for granted or ignores the gifts that God bestowed upon every person. Some gifts may appear underutilized, yet the gift is uniquely possessed. Human integrity stands atop all gifts bestowed by the creator. A good nurse preserves the gift of human integrity through deliberately acknowledging the worth of every person whose life is touched during a nursing encounter."

DIANN WALKER WILLIAMS, MSN, RN, CNE
Vice President for Institutional Effectiveness
Nursing & Allied Health
Southeast Arkansas College
Pine Bluff, AR
Expertise:
Nursing Education Administration
Medical Surgical Nursing
Education:
University of Arkansas- Pine Bluff (BSN)
St. Louis University (MSN)

    ❝ Know that every patient you encounter is the unique creation of our God; treat them as if they are our Lord himself."

"Be most attentive to those intuitive nudgings and subtle feelings; they are much more reliable than your logical thought."

NANCY B. WILLIAMSON, RN, PHD
Retired from Medical College of Georgia
Augusta, GA
Expertise:
Health Care Program Development and Evaluation
Education:
Wichita St. Joseph School of Nursing
Medical College of Georgia
Georgia State University

“ My favorite professional book, J. Welch's, *Winning* (2005, New York: Harper Collins Publishers, Inc.) is the inspiration for many of my words of wisdom below.”

On employment:

“Find the right job for you and you'll never really work again. (There are so many options in the nursing profession that there is a 'perfect' job for everyone).

Nothing will get you a new job faster than terrific performance in your old one.

Contribute your knowledge, expertise, and skills to your environment.

When you have stopped learning in your current position, it is time to find a new one.”

On hiring:

“The wrong person is worse than no person.

Hire the best people that you can and then get out of their way.”

On happiness:

“Happiness is a choice. Decide to be happy in whatever circumstances you find yourself.”

On administration:

"Communicate clearly & calmly.

Say what you mean; mean what you say.

Do not be afraid of or avoid conflict; it usually leads to better decisions."

On nursing academia:

"To be successful in academia, do not consider employment a job. Rather it is a career & may eventually progress to a lifestyle."

CAROLYN B. YUCHA, RN, PhD, FAAN
Dean, Schools of Nursing and Allied Health Sciences
University of Nevada, Las Vegas
Las Vegas, NV
Expertise:
Academic Administration
Nursing Administration
Writing for Publication
Research Interests:
Stress Reduction
Non-Pharmacological Treatment of Hypertension
Nursing Education
Education:
State University of New York at Albany (BS in Nursing)
State University of New York at Buffalo (MS in Adult
    Health Nursing)
Upstate Medical Center (PhD in Physiology)

❝ My favorite two phrases that I use, I learned over time and do not know who originated them, but I appreciate their truth:

'With repetition comes comfort.'

I use this phrase in the clinical settings for students as they struggle to be 'flawless' in their rotations. They become easily frustrated as they begin to learn their own 'style' of nursing. As they do skills repetitiously, I see the growth and comfort in their efforts.

'If you have to make up a story to get to your answer, it's not the right answer.'

I use this phrase for students who are taking multiple choice exams. Students commonly assume things in questions and I frequently remind them that everything I wanted for them to know in the question is there, no more, no less. Many students look at the answers before reading the question. I encourage them to read the question first, then answer without looking at the options, then see if one of the options matches their own answer."

Zelne Zamora, DNP, RN

Assistant Professor
Course Coordinator
Nursing Pharmacology and Adult Health I
Loma Linda University School of Nursing
Loma Linda, CA

Expertise:
Medical Surgical Nursing in Surgical Units Specializing
in Orthopedics, Urology, Plastic Surgery and Bariatrics

Education:
Loma Linda University School of Nursing (BS)
Azusa Pacific University (MS)
University of San Diego (DNP)

Some things you may not encounter for your whole life, but it is always good to have some information at hand, so you may be able to help people out some day in a certain way."

"When something serious happens, people tend initially to avoid. As a professional nurse as well as a sincere person, you can empower them. It is important to get them actively involved in their surgical intervention."

JUN ZHANG, PhD
Assistant Professor
Seton Hall College of Nursing
South Orange, NJ
Expertise:
Gerontological Issues
Maternal and Child Health Nursing
Advanced Research Issues
Advanced Nursing Issues
Nursing Education
Education:
University of Pennsylvania

" It is important never to lose our passion for helping others or caring about those less fortunate than ourselves. It is the act of reaching out and creating connections within humanity or nature that gives us meaning as human beings and enriches our identity as nurses."

"It is important to recognize what we know and what we don't know—and then go look it up in the literature or consult another specialist."

ELKE JONES ZSCHAEBITZ, MSN, FNP-BC
Instructor
University of Virginia School of Nursing
Clinician/Nurse Practitioner
High Risk Breast and Ovarian Cancer Program
UVA Health System
Charlottesville, VA
Expertise:
Rural Health Care in Global Settings of Health Disparity
Telehealth/Telenursing
Women's Health/Primary Care
Education:
Villanova University (BSN)
Midwestern State University (MSN)

LaVergne, TN USA
30 March 2011
222089LV00001B/10/P